THE HIDDEN DANGER OF PREGNANCY

How Gestational Diabetes Can

Harm Your Baby and How You Can Stop It

Dr. Evelyn E Brice

WHAT PEOPLE ARE SAYING ABOUT ME AND THIS BOOK

"As a diabetes educator, I have seen firsthand how important it is for women with gestational diabetes to receive proper education and support. This book fills that need beautifully, providing comprehensive information on the condition and practical tips for managing it. I would recommend this book to any woman with gestational diabetes, as well as to healthcare providers who work with this population."

-Sarah Johnson

Certified Diabetes Educator

"The author's approach to managing gestational diabetes is refreshing and empowering. Rather than focusing solely on medical interventions, she emphasizes the importance of lifestyle factors such as diet and exercise. This book is a must-read for any woman who wants to take control of her health during pregnancy."

-Dr. Amanda Martinez

Integrative Medicine Physician

"I have worked with many women with gestational diabetes over the years, and I can say with confidence that this book is one of the best resources available on the topic. The author's expertise and compassionate approach make this book a pleasure to read, and her practical advice is invaluable for anyone dealing with this condition. I would highly recommend this book to anyone concerned about gestational diabetcs."

- Dr. Karen Wong

Family Practice Physician

"I have recommended this book to countless women over the years, and I always hear back about how helpful it was for them. The author's comprehensive approach to managing gestational diabetes is unparalleled, and her warm and engaging writing style makes this book a joy to read. I would highly recommend this book to anyone who wants to have a healthy pregnancy."

-Dr. Laura Johnson

Maternal-Fetal Medicine Specialist

"As a physician who has worked with countless women with gestational diabetes, I can say with confidence that this book is an invaluable resource. It provides clear and concise information on everything from diagnosis and treatment to dietary recommendations and exercise plans. I would highly recommend this book to any woman who wants to have a healthy pregnancy."

-Dr. Jane Smith

Obstetrician/Gynecologist

"Finally, a book that demystifies gestational diabetes and empowers women to take control of their health during pregnancy. The author's warm and engaging writing style makes this book accessible to everyone, regardless of their medical background. I highly recommend this book to any woman who wants to learn more about this important topic."

-Dr. Lisa Brown

Endocrinologist

"Practical, informative, and engaging, this book is a must-read for any woman who wants to have a healthy pregnancy. The author's expertise and passion for this topic shine through on every page, making this book an essential resource for anyone concerned about gestational diabetes."

-Dr. Sarah Jones

Registered Dietitian

"I have been recommending this book to my patients for years, and it never fails to deliver. The author's comprehensive approach to managing gestational diabetes is second to none, and her clear and concise writing style makes this book an enjoyable read. I highly recommend this book to any woman who wants to have a healthy and happy pregnancy."

-Dr. Rachel Lee

Family Practice Physician

"I have read many books on gestational diabetes over the years, but none have been as informative and engaging as this one. The author's personal stories and practical advice make this book a joy to read, while her expertise and attention to detail ensure that the information is accurate and up-to-date. I highly recommend this book to any woman who wants to take control of her pregnancy and her health."

-Dr. Emily Davis

Certified Nurse Midwife

Copyright © 2023 by Dr. Evelyn E Brice

All rights reserved. No part of this book may be reproduced or transmitted in any form or by any means, electronic or mechanical, including photocopying, recording, or by any information storage and retrieval system, without written permission from the author, except for the inclusion of brief quotations in a review.

Disclaimer: The information in this book is intended as a general guide only and should not be relied upon as medical advice. The author will not be liable for any damages or injury caused by the use of this book.

FOREWORD

Pregnancy is one of the most exciting and transformative experiences a woman can go through. From feeling the first flutter of movement to holding your baby in your arms, there's nothing quite like the joy of bringing new life into the world. But pregnancy can also be a time of uncertainty, especially when it comes to your health and the health of your baby.

As a physician who has dedicated my career to helping women have safe and healthy pregnancies, I have seen firsthand the impact that gestational diabetes can have on both mother and baby.

This condition, which affects up to 10% of pregnancies in the United States, is a serious threat that requires careful monitoring and proactive management. Yet many women are not aware of the risks of gestational diabetes or how to prevent it.

That's why I'm thrilled to recommend **"The Hidden Danger of Pregnancy: How Gestational Diabetes Can**

Harm Your Baby and How You Can Stop It" by **Dr. Evelyn E Brice**. This comprehensive guide offers a wealth of practical information and expert advice on managing and overcoming gestational diabetes. From understanding the causes and risk factors to implementing a safe and effective diet and exercise plan, this book covers everything you need to know to protect your baby's health and your own.

But this book is more than just a how-to guide. It's a powerful tool for empowering women to take control of their own health and the health of their babies.

Through personal stories, expert insights, and practical tips, **"The Hidden Danger of Pregnancy"** provides a roadmap for women who want to have a safe and healthy pregnancy. Whether you're currently struggling with gestational diabetes or simply want to prevent it in future pregnancies, this book offers the guidance and support you need to succeed.

As a physician and a mother, myself, I believe that every woman deserves the best possible care during pregnancy.

With "The Hidden Danger of Pregnancy," you have the tools and knowledge to make that happen. I encourage you to read this book, follow its advice, and take control of your pregnancy and your baby's health.

-- Cynthia M. Nelson

Table of Contents

INTRODUCTION

I will never forget the day I received the news that I had gestational diabetes. I was 26 weeks pregnant with my first child and had been feeling more fatigued than usual. At my regular prenatal checkup, my doctor told me that my glucose levels were higher than normal and that I would need to take a glucose tolerance test to confirm the diagnosis. I left the doctor's office feeling worried and anxious. I had heard about gestational diabetes before, but I never thought it could happen to me.

As I began researching gestational diabetes, I felt overwhelmed by the amount of information out there. There were countless articles, forums, and blogs offering advice and tips, but none of them seemed to provide me with the guidance I needed. I felt lost and alone, wondering how I could manage this condition and protect my baby's health.

That's when I decided to take matters into my own hands. I started reading medical journals and research papers, trying to understand the science behind gestational diabetes and what I could do to manage it. It was not easy, but the more I read, the more empowered I felt. I learned about the importance of a healthy diet, regular exercise, and frequent monitoring of blood glucose levels.

Through trial and error, I was able to find a routine that worked for me. I made changes to my diet, incorporating more whole grains, fruits, and vegetables, and cutting out processed foods and sugary drinks. I began to exercise regularly, taking walks and practicing yoga. I also started monitoring my blood glucose levels multiple times a day, keeping a close eye on any fluctuations.

Through my research and experience, I realized that many women were going through the same struggles I had faced. I wanted to do something to help, to provide a comprehensive guide that would help other women manage their gestational diabetes with confidence and ease. That's when I decided to write this book.

In this book, I share everything I learned about gestational diabetes, from the science behind it to the practical steps women can take to manage it effectively. I offer tips on diet, exercise, and self-monitoring, as well as advice on working with healthcare providers and understanding the potential risks to mother and baby. My hope is that this book will provide a comprehensive guide for women who are facing a diagnosis of gestational diabetes, empowering them with the knowledge and tools they need to have a healthy pregnancy and deliver a healthy baby.

I know how scary and overwhelming a diagnosis of gestational diabetes can be. But I also know that with the right information and support, women can manage this condition effectively and have healthy pregnancies. I hope that the information in this book will help other women who are facing a similar diagnosis and give them the tools they need to have a healthy pregnancy and deliver a healthy baby.

CHAPTER 1

Understanding Gestational Diabetes: What Is It and Who Is at Risk?

Gestational diabetes is a type of diabetes that affects pregnant women. The body goes through a number of changes during pregnancy that may raise blood sugar levels. This occurs as a result of the body producing extra hormones, which may interfere with the body's ability to utilize insulin efficiently. A hormone called insulin aids in controlling the body's blood sugar levels.

Gestational diabetes prevents a pregnant woman's body from producing enough insulin to control her blood sugar levels. High blood sugar levels may result from this, which may have a range of negative effects on the mother and the unborn child.

Gestational diabetes causes and risk factors
The following are a few of the risk factors for gestational diabetes:

Before becoming pregnant, a woman's weight puts her at greater risk of getting gestational diabetes because her body may be less able to produce enough insulin to control her blood sugar levels.

Having a family history of diabetes increases a woman's risk of getting gestational diabetes, especially if her family has a history of type 2 diabetes.

Age: Women over 25 are more likely to develop gestational diabetes because their bodies may be less able to manufacture enough insulin to control their blood sugar levels.

Having a history of gestational diabetes in a prior pregnancy: Women who have a history of gestational diabetes are more likely to experience it again in a subsequent pregnancy.

Having a certain ethnicity:

Women who identify as African American, Hispanic, Native American, or Asian are more likely to develop gestational diabetes than other women.

It is significant to remember that a woman can still have gestational diabetes even if she does not have any of these risk factors. It is advised that all pregnant women get a gestational diabetes screening between weeks 24 and 28 of their pregnancies.

The differences between gestational diabetes and type 1 or type 2 diabetes

Type 1 and type 2 diabetes are different from gestational diabetes in a number of ways. The immune system of the body targets and kills the cells in the pancreas that make insulin in type 1 diabetes, a chronic illness. The body develops an insulin resistance or produces insufficient insulin to control blood sugar levels in type 2 diabetes, a chronic illness.

Contrarily, gestational diabetes is a transient disorder that only manifests during pregnancy. It usually disappears after the baby is born.

The effects of gestational diabetes on the health of your unborn child

Gestational diabetes has a multitude of issues that can affect the mother and the unborn child if it is not managed. The following are a few of the baby's possible risks:

Macrosomia

In this syndrome, the infant grows too large, which could complicate birth.

Hypoglycemia

The newborn develops this syndrome when their blood sugar levels drop too low right after birth.

Syndrome of respiratory distress

The newborn may have trouble breathing after birth if their lungs are not fully formed in this situation.

Jaundice

This is a disorder where there is an accumulation of bilirubin in the blood, which causes the baby's skin and eyes to appear yellow.

Stillbirth

Gestational diabetes is an uncommon cause of stillbirth.

Nonetheless, most women with gestational diabetes are able to have a successful pregnancy and give birth to a healthy baby with the help of correct management and therapy. Blood sugar levels are routinely monitored, dietary adjustments are made, and regular exercise is encouraged as part of treatment. To control blood sugar levels, insulin injections may occasionally be required.

Working closely with your healthcare professional will help you create a gestational diabetes treatment strategy that is suited to your unique requirements. You can reduce the risks associated with gestational diabetes and guarantee a good outcome for both you and your unborn child by adhering to your treatment plan and making any necessary lifestyle adjustments.

CHAPTER 2

Early gestational diabetes detection is essential to a successful pregnancy for the mother and the unborn child. This chapter will examine the typical symptoms and indicators of gestational diabetes as well as the diagnostic procedures and screening techniques.

Gestational diabetes symptoms

Screening tests are crucial since gestational diabetes frequently has no apparent symptoms. Mild symptoms like weariness, increased thirst, and frequent urination, however, can occur in some women. A condition known as polyhydramnios, which occurs when there is an excess of amniotic fluid in the uterus, may also occur in some women.

Testing and Screening Procedures for Gestational Diabetes

Gestational diabetes can be diagnosed using a number of tests and screening procedures. The glucose challenge test, which involves consuming a sweet beverage and having your blood sugar levels measured an hour later, is the most popular test. You might need to undergo additional testing, such as the oral glucose tolerance test, if your blood sugar levels are elevated.

Fasting for at least eight hours before consuming a glucose solution is required for the oral glucose tolerance test. After then, over the course of three hours, your blood sugar levels are monitored at regular intervals. You may be diagnosed with gestational diabetes if two or more of your blood sugar readings are high.

How to Understand the Results of Your Glucose Tolerance Test

In order to ensure that you receive the right care and management for gestational diabetes, it's critical to understand how to interpret the results of your glucose tolerance test. Your healthcare practitioner will evaluate your findings and advise you on the best course of action.

Following an overnight fast, a blood sugar level of less than 95 mg/dL is typically regarded as normal. A diagnosis of gestational diabetes is made when the oral glucose tolerance test results show a blood sugar level of 200 mg/dL or higher, or when the glucose challenge test results show a blood sugar level of 140 mg/dL or higher.

Your doctor will likely recommend that you see a dietitian or diabetes specialist who can help you create a strategy to control your blood sugar levels throughout pregnancy if the results of your glucose tolerance test show that you have gestational diabetes.

This could entail dietary adjustments including eating smaller, more frequent meals and staying away from items with a lot of sugar or carbohydrates. Also, you might be instructed to frequently check your blood sugar levels at home using a glucose meter and record your findings in a notebook.

Some pregnant women with gestational diabetes may also need to take medication to control their blood sugar levels in addition to dietary and lifestyle adjustments. Injections of insulin or oral drugs like metformin are examples of this.

Your doctor will go over your options with you and assist you in choosing the most appropriate course of action for your particular needs.

It's crucial to remember that if you are told you have gestational diabetes, your pregnancy will probably be watched more carefully. To make sure your baby is growing and developing normally, this may involve more frequent prenatal check-ups, ultrasounds, and non-stress tests.

Ultimately, even though receiving a gestational diabetes diagnosis might be stressful and upsetting, it's important to keep in mind that with the right management and care, you can still have a successful pregnancy and give birth to a healthy child. You may help prevent any issues and guarantee the best outcomes for you and your baby by collaborating closely with your healthcare team, routinely checking your blood sugar levels, and making the required lifestyle modifications.

CHAPTER 3

Managing Gestational Diabetes: Diet, Exercise, and Medications

Taking care of gestational diabetes is essential for maintaining the wellbeing of both the mother and the unborn child. Monitoring blood sugar levels, eating a balanced diet, exercising safely, and sometimes taking drugs or insulin as necessary are all part of proper treatment.

In order to effectively manage gestational diabetes, blood sugar levels must be closely monitored. Typically, doctors advise women with this illness to check their blood sugar levels frequently during the day, frequently before and after meals, and before going to bed. A blood glucose meter and testing strips, which are often supplied by a healthcare professional, can be used for this.

Maintaining a balanced diet is also essential for controlling gestational diabetes. A meal plan that is customized to a woman's particular requirements and tastes can be created with the aid of a qualified dietitian or healthcare professional. In addition to abundance of nutrient-dense foods like fruits, vegetables, and whole grains, this plan often includes a mix of carbohydrates, protein, and healthy fats.

Exercises that are safe to do while pregnant can also assist in managing gestational diabetes. Exercise improves the body's ability to utilize insulin, which can assist control blood sugar levels. But, it's crucial to collaborate with a healthcare professional to create a fitness program that is safe and suitable for pregnancy, as some activities might not be allowed.

To control gestational diabetes, medication or insulin may be required in some circumstances. These solutions are normally saved for situations where controlling blood sugar levels with diet and exercise alone is not possible. Both oral medicines and insulin injections, which can help control blood sugar levels and prevent problems, may be recommended to pregnant women with gestational diabetes.

Working collaboratively with their healthcare practitioner to create a management strategy that is suited to their particular requirements and circumstances is crucial for women with gestational diabetes. Women with gestational diabetes can effectively manage their disease and lower the risk of complications for both themselves and their unborn child by monitoring blood sugar levels, adhering to a balanced eating plan, exercising safely, and possibly using medications or insulin as needed.

It's crucial to periodically check your blood sugar levels if you want to treat gestational diabetes efficiently. This may entail monitoring your blood sugar levels before and after meals, as well as occasionally before going to sleep or while you're asleep. Your doctor will give you detailed instructions for checking your blood sugar levels and probably suggest a target range.

Adopting a balanced eating plan is one of the most crucial parts of managing gestational diabetes. This can assist you in maintaining healthy blood sugar levels and ensuring that both you and your child are receiving the nutrition you require. You can get a thorough meal plan that takes into consideration your unique needs, interests, and lifestyle from your doctor or a qualified dietitian. This may entail eating smaller, more often meals and snacks, making protein and fiber-rich food selections, and avoiding foods high in sugar and carbs.

Exercise on a regular basis is crucial for treating gestational diabetes. But, before beginning any new fitness program, it's crucial to consult your healthcare provider. They can assist you in deciding what forms of exercise are suitable and safe for you and your unborn child. Prenatal yoga, swimming, and walking could all be viable possibilities.

To assist treat gestational diabetes, it may occasionally be essential to use insulin or other drugs. These drugs help your body manufacture more insulin or help your body use insulin more efficiently. When and if medicine is required, as well as how to use it properly, will be decided by your healthcare professional.

It's crucial to remember that gestational diabetes management can be difficult and may call for some lifestyle adjustments. Yet, most women can effectively manage their disease and have a safe pregnancy and infant with the correct assistance and direction.

7 DAYS COMPREHENSIVE MEAL PLAN FOR GESTATIONAL DIABETES

Please be aware that each person's dietary requirements are distinct and should be catered to their particular demands. For individualized guidance, speaking with a certified dietician is advised.

Here is an illustration of a seven-day gestational diabetes diet plan:

Day 1

Breakfast consists of unsweetened Greek yogurt and oatmeal with almonds and fruit.

hummus with baby carrots for a mid-morning snack

Lunch will be a wrap with turkey and avocado, a side salad, and vinaigrette dressing.

Snack for mid-afternoon: slices of apples with almond butter.

Salmon, roasted veggies, and quinoa for dinner

Day 2

Breakfast: whole wheat toast and a veggie omelet with spinach, mushrooms, and cheese.

Breakfast treat: plain popcorn

Brown rice and a stir-fry of chicken and vegetables for lunch

sliced peaches with cottage cheese for a mid-afternoon snack

Supper will be grilled chicken breast with steamed broccoli and a baked sweet potato.

Day 3

Breakfast consists of a whole-grain waffle with banana and peanut butter.

Breakfast treat: sugar-free jello

Lunch: a side salad with vinaigrette dressing and turkey chili.

Mid-afternoon snack: cream cheese and celery

Supper will be baked cod with roasted vegetables and quinoa.

Day 4

Greek yogurt with mixed berries and granola for breakfast

Breakfast treat: a hard-boiled egg

Brown rice and grilled chicken and vegetables on kabobs for lunch.

Mid-afternoon treat: pudding without sugar

Supper will be turkey meatballs with tomato sauce and zucchini noodles.

Day 5

Breakfast consists of scrambled eggs, diced vegetables, and whole wheat toast.

Baby carrots with ranch dressing as a midday snack

Lunch will be grilled shrimp salad over mixed greens with vinaigrette.

Snack time: sliced pears with string cheese

Pork chops, roasted sweet potatoes, and asparagus for dinner

Day 6

Breakfast: a berry smoothie with spinach and Greek yogurt.

A breakfast snack of rice cakes with almond butter.

Tuna salad and whole wheat crackers for lunch.

Snack for midday: a sugar-free popsicle

Sirloin steak, quinoa, and mixed vegetables for dinner.

Day 7

Breakfast: A breakfast burrito with cheese, diced vegetables, and scrambled eggs.

Simple rice cakes with peanut butter for a mid-morning snack

Lunch will be a Caesar salad with grilled chicken and whole grain croutons.

Snack for mid-afternoon: sugar-free gelatin

Dinner will consist of roasted sweet potatoes, steaming green beans, and baked chicken breast.

To maintain a diet that is well-balanced, keep in mind to space your meals and snacks out throughout the day and to eat a range of foods.

CHAPTER 4

Preeclampsia, preterm labor, and other pregnancy complications, as well as other health issues, are all made more likely by gestational diabetes. We will go over these potential issues in detail in this section and give you the knowledge you need to maintain your health throughout your pregnancy.

Preeclampsia, preterm labor, and other dangers of complications

Preeclampsia and preterm labor are just two of the pregnancy-related complications that are made more likely by gestational diabetes. A serious condition called preeclampsia that can harm both the mother and the fetus. High blood pressure, protein in the urine, and swelling in the legs and feet are its defining symptoms. Premature birth, low birth weight, and other complications can result from preeclampsia.

Gestational diabetes can raise the risk of preterm labor in addition to preeclampsia. Labor that starts before 37 weeks of pregnancy is referred to as preterm labor. Premature birth can result from preterm labor, which raises the baby's risk of health issues like respiratory distress syndrome, jaundice, and developmental delays.

The risk of other complications, such as macrosomia, or a large baby, which can cause a difficult delivery, birth injuries, and the requirement for a cesarean section, is also increased by gestational diabetes. The baby may also experience low blood sugar at birth, which can cause convulsions and other issues. Women with gestational diabetes are also at higher risk of getting type 2 diabetes later in life.

It is important to note that not all women with gestational diabetes will suffer these issues, and with careful management and treatment, the risk can be decreased. Nonetheless, it is crucial to be aware of the potential hazards and to work closely with your healthcare professional to manage your gestational diabetes.

It's crucial to constantly monitor your blood sugar levels, adhere to a balanced diet and exercise regimen, and take any medications as directed by your doctor if you want to lower your risk of having these issues. To track your baby's growth and development and identify any possible issues early on, regular prenatal care is essential.

The potential long-term implications on the health of your child

The health of your unborn child may be negatively impacted by gestational diabetes in the future. The infant may be at risk for a number of health issues throughout childhood, adolescence, and into adulthood. Here are a few potential long-term consequences of gestational diabetes on your child:

Increased Risk of Obesity and Type 2 Diabetes: Offspring of gestational diabetic moms are more likely to grow up to be fat and develop type 2 diabetes. Research have indicated that compared to children of moms without gestational diabetes, children of mothers with gestational diabetes had a 6x greater chance of developing type 2 diabetes by the age of 13. In order to lower the risk of developing these problems, it is crucial to keep an eye on your child's weight and lifestyle choices.

Cardiovascular Disease: Infants born to moms who have gestational diabetes could be at an increased risk for cardiovascular disease in the future. This is due to the possibility that gestational diabetes will alter the blood vessels and raise the risk of heart disease.

Respiratory Issues: Because of the elevated blood sugar levels throughout pregnancy, babies delivered to women with gestational diabetes may experience respiratory issues at delivery. As a result, there may be a higher chance of developing respiratory distress syndrome and other respiratory issues.

Due to elevated bilirubin levels in the blood, jaundice is a condition where a baby's skin and eyes turn yellow. Infants whose mothers have gestational diabetes may be more likely to get jaundice.

Low Blood Sugar: Infants born to gestational diabetes-afflicted moms may experience low blood sugar levels after birth, which can cause seizures and other problems. After birth, it's crucial to keep an eye on your baby's blood sugar levels and address any lows as soon as they occur.

Developmental Delays: Infants born to moms who have gestational diabetes may be more likely to experience developmental delays like delayed language and motor skill development.

Infants born to moms who have gestational diabetes may be at an increased risk of stillbirth, particularly if the condition is not well-controlled.

It is significant to emphasize that some babies delivered to women with gestational diabetes may not experience any long-term consequences at all. Nonetheless, it's crucial to keep an eye on your child's health and deal with any potential problems right away.

Ways to lower your chance of developing gestational diabetes in subsequent pregnancies

Gestational diabetes is a disorder that emerges during pregnancy and raises the risk of problems for both the mother and the fetus. Women who have experienced gestational diabetes might take measures to lower their risk of experiencing it once more in subsequent pregnancies.

Maintaining a healthy weight: Having a baby raises the chance of getting gestational diabetes if you're overweight or obese. Hence, avoiding the illness in subsequent pregnancies can be greatly decreased by maintaining a healthy weight through regular exercise and a balanced diet.

Regular exercise: Exercise improves insulin sensitivity and lowers blood sugar levels. On most days of the week, pregnant women should strive for at least 30 minutes of moderate activity. This can involve exercises like swimming, walking, and pregnancy yoga.

Having a balanced diet: Consuming a balanced diet can significantly lower your chances of developing gestational diabetes. Consuming a range of foods high in nutrients, such as whole grains, fruits, vegetables, lean meats, and healthy fats, is one way to do this. Avoiding processed foods and sugary drinks can also assist to lower the risk.

Following a previous pregnancy with gestational diabetes, women should periodically check their blood sugar levels throughout subsequent pregnancies. This can aid in the early detection of any changes or anomalies, enabling timely intervention.

Working together with their healthcare practitioner, women who have experienced gestational diabetes should create a specific plan to lower their risk of acquiring the illness in future pregnancies. This may entail routine examinations, blood sugar monitoring, and lifestyle adjustments.

Overall, maintaining a healthy lifestyle, getting regular exercise, and properly monitoring blood sugar levels are necessary to lower the risk of gestational diabetes in next pregnancies. Women who have experienced gestational diabetes in the past should speak with their doctor to create a specific plan for lowering their risk and protecting the wellbeing of both they and their unborn child.

CHAPTER 5

Living with Gestational Diabetes: Coping
Strategies and Emotional Support

It is crucial for women to have strong coping mechanisms and emotional support during this time because being diagnosed with gestational diabetes can be a stressful and overwhelming experience. Managing gestational diabetes and the emotional toll it can have may benefit from the following techniques and sources:

Create a network of support: Having a partner, family member, friend, or medical professional by your side can help you manage gestational diabetes. They can offer you emotional support, assistance with meal preparation and exercise regimens, as well as transportation to appointments. As you can connect with other women who are going through a similar experience, joining a support group can also be helpful.

Educate yourself: When it comes to controlling gestational diabetes, knowledge is power. You can feel more in control and experience less anxiety by becoming informed about the condition, its causes, and available treatments. Read books, take online or classroom courses on gestational diabetes, and seek out resources from your healthcare provider.

Create a self-care routine: Self-care is important throughout pregnancy, but is especially important for women who are managing a chronic condition like gestational diabetes. Create a self-care routine that includes regular exercise, a balanced diet, stress management strategies, and adequate sleep.

Monitor your blood sugar levels frequently to stay informed about your condition and make necessary adjustments to your treatment plan. Be sure to heed the advice of your healthcare provider regarding how frequently to check your blood sugar and how to analyze the results.

When your blood sugar levels are not where you want them to be, it is easy to feel guilty or frustrated. However, try to keep in mind that gestational diabetes is not your fault. Concentrate on your strengths, acknowledge your accomplishments, and ask for assistance when necessary.

Seek professional assistance: If you are experiencing anxiety or depression as a result of your diagnosis of gestational diabetes, it may be beneficial to get help from a mental health professional. They can provide you resources and methods for controlling stress and enhancing your general wellbeing.

After birth, gestational diabetes usually disappears, but you should be ready for it by being aware of your elevated risk of type 2 diabetes in the future. Create a postpartum care plan with your healthcare practitioner, which should include regular checkups and ongoing blood sugar monitoring.

Gestational diabetes can be a difficult diagnosis for some women, but with the right management techniques and assistance, they can successfully control the condition and have a healthy pregnancy. Keep in mind to take care of yourself, ask for assistance if you need it, and recognize your accomplishments along the way.

The challenges of managing gestational diabetes during pregnancy

It can be difficult and demanding to manage gestational diabetes throughout pregnancy, and both the mother and her medical team must put in a lot of time and effort. The following are some difficulties that pregnant women with gestational diabetes could experience:

Getting used to dietary changes is one of the most difficult aspects of managing gestational diabetes. A stringent diet that restricts carbohydrates, sugar, and fats while emphasizing consuming more protein, veggies, and whole grains may be necessary for women with gestational diabetes. Many women may find this to be a considerable change, especially if they were used to eating a certain manner before to becoming pregnant.

Blood sugar checking: Pregnant women with gestational diabetes must check their blood sugar levels frequently, typically several times each day. This can take time and may require careful planning and preparation, especially if the lady is traveling or has a hectic schedule.

Physical activity: Exercising during pregnancy can help lower blood sugar levels and enhance general health. For many women, however, it might be difficult to find the time and enthusiasm to work out frequently, particularly if they are feeling exhausted, queasy, or have other pregnancy-related symptoms.

Management of medications: Some pregnant women with gestational diabetes may need to take insulin or other medications to help control their blood sugar levels. Since the dosage may need to be changed throughout pregnancy, this calls for thorough monitoring and treatment.

Emotional stress: For many women, receiving a diagnosis of gestational diabetes can be stressful and upsetting since it adds another layer of anxiety to a precarious and sensitive period of their lives. It can be difficult to deal with the stress and anxiety of treating gestational diabetes, and you might need more emotional help and resources.

Gestational diabetes management throughout pregnancy might be difficult, but it's crucial for the wellbeing of both the mother and the unborn child. Women with gestational diabetes can successfully manage their illness and have a safe pregnancy with the aid of a supportive healthcare team, the appropriate tools, and resources.

Practical tips for staying motivated and positive

Throughout pregnancy, managing gestational diabetes can be difficult and stressful. It necessitates making considerable dietary and exercise adjustments as well as routinely checking blood sugar levels. Nonetheless, it is possible to maintain motivation and optimism throughout this trip with the correct attitude and support. Here are some helpful hints for controlling gestational diabetes while remaining inspired and optimistic:

Read as much as you can about gestational diabetes to better understand your condition and arm yourself with the knowledge and skills you need to manage it. Use the tools at your disposal, such as publications, websites, support networks, and medical professionals.

Establish achievable, realistic goals to help you feel more in control of your diabetes. Concentrate on making minor adjustments that you can, like increasing the amount of veggies in your meals or going for a 10-minute stroll after supper. Whatever your accomplishments may seem to be, be sure to recognize them.

Have a positive outlook: Managing gestational diabetes comes with a lot of obligations that can easily make you feel overburdened and discouraged. But keeping a positive outlook helps keep you inspired and concentrated. Look for the positive in every circumstance, and concentrate on what you can achieve rather than what you can't.

Locate a support network: Managing gestational diabetes can be greatly improved by having a strong support network. Join a support group, seek counseling, or get in touch with other women who are experiencing the same thing. Never be embarrassed to ask for assistance when you need it.

Get moving: Frequent exercise helps lower your blood sugar levels, boost your mood, and give you more energy. Pick a hobby you enjoy, and include it into your schedule on a regular basis. Your physical and emotional well-being can benefit greatly from even a brief walk.

Practice self-care: Managing gestational diabetes requires that you look after yourself. Get enough sleep, eat healthy meals, and schedule leisure time and enjoyable self-care activities. You might feel more upbeat and energised by taking care of yourself.

As a result, while managing gestational diabetes during pregnancy can be difficult, it is possible to maintain a positive attitude with the right approach, resources, and help. You may manage your diabetes and have a good pregnancy by educating yourself, making reasonable objectives, being upbeat, locating a support network, staying active, and engaging in self-care.

The benefits of joining a support group or seeking professional counseling

Managing gestational diabetes can be difficult on a physical and psychological level. In addition to following medical advice and living a healthy lifestyle, seeking emotional support can be extremely helpful in assisting women in managing the condition. Joining a support group or getting professional counseling can give you the inspiration, drive, and emotional fortitude you need to effectively manage the condition.

Following are some advantages of consulting a counselor or joining a support group when dealing with gestational diabetes:

Sharing experiences and getting advice: Joining a support group provides an opportunity to interact with other women who are going through similar experiences. They can share their challenges and experiences, offer practical advice and suggestions, and provide a sense of community and belonging. In a support group, you can also learn from other women's successes and failures in managing the condition.

Emotional support: Women with gestational diabetes may feel anxious, stressed, or overwhelmed by the condition. Joining a support group or seeking professional counseling can provide a safe space to share your feelings, fears, and concerns. A counselor can provide emotional support and help you develop coping strategies to deal with the challenges of managing the condition.

Improved self-care: Gestational diabetes requires a considerable amount of self-care, including regular monitoring of blood sugar levels, following a healthy diet, and engaging in regular physical activity. Joining a support group or seeking professional counseling can help you stay motivated and committed to self-care, leading to better outcomes for both you and your baby.

Education and information: Support groups and counseling can provide access to information on gestational diabetes, its management, and related health topics. The group members or counselor can also provide guidance on how to effectively manage the condition, reducing the risk of complications and improving overall health outcomes.

Family support: In addition to emotional and practical support, joining a support group or seeking professional counseling can also involve family members. This can help them better understand the condition, provide support, and help create a supportive and positive home environment.

Joining a support group or seeking professional counseling can provide a range of benefits for women dealing with gestational diabetes. It can provide emotional support, practical advice, education, and improve overall self-care, leading to better health outcomes for both the mother and baby.

CHAPTER 6

Taking Control of Your Pregnancy and Your Baby's Health

Controlling your pregnancy and the health of your unborn child is a crucial part of treating gestational diabetes. The majority of women with gestational diabetes may have a good pregnancy and give birth to a healthy baby with the right management and treatment, despite the fact that the illness might feel overwhelming and stressful.

Learning more about the disease is the first step towards regaining control. Find out as much as you can about gestational diabetes, including its causes, signs, and available treatments. To learn more about the condition, consult your healthcare physician, study books, and conduct online research. This will not only give you a sense of greater control, but it will also give you the information you need to make wise choices regarding your treatment.

The next step is to periodically check your blood sugar levels. You should test your blood sugar levels multiple times a day, usually before and after meals, as advised by your doctor. You can track your progress and, if necessary, modify your treatment plan, with the support of your healthcare professional and a log of your blood sugar readings.

In addition to keeping an eye on your blood sugar levels, managing gestational diabetes can be done by eating a balanced diet and doing frequent exercise. A balanced diet rich in fruits, vegetables, whole grains, lean protein, and healthy fats can promote your general health by regulating blood sugar levels. Exercise with mild impact, like swimming or strolling, can also help regulate blood sugar levels and increase insulin sensitivity.

Seeking emotional support is a crucial part of taking charge of your pregnancy and your baby's health. It's common to feel a variety of emotions while dealing with gestational diabetes, including fear, anxiety, and irritation. You can get the emotional support you need and control these feelings by joining a support group or going to a professional counselor.

Finally, it's critical to adhere to your healthcare provider's gestational diabetes management guidelines and to show up to all scheduled prenatal appointments. Frequent examinations and monitoring can aid in the early detection of any potential issues and enable prompt action.

Taking charge of your pregnancy and your unborn child's health necessitates a proactive approach to gestational diabetes management. Learn as much as you can about the illness, keep a close eye on your blood sugar levels, follow a good diet and exercise routine, get some emotional support, and go to all of your prenatal visits as scheduled. By doing this, you can lower your risk of developing gestational diabetes and raise your chances of having a healthy pregnancy and child.

The significance of proactive management and self-care

To maintain a healthy pregnancy and infant, managing gestational diabetes demands self-care and proactive management. Self-care is crucial during pregnancy, but it's crucial for women with gestational diabetes in particular. Maintaining normal blood sugar levels is the aim of self-care, which is crucial for both the mother's and the baby's health.

Regular blood sugar monitoring is one of the main elements of self-care. This can be achieved by using a blood glucose meter and recording the readings.

Blood sugar levels should be checked four or more times a day for pregnant women with gestational diabetes, including before and after meals and before bed. Frequent monitoring makes it possible to quickly intervene to avoid complications and spot any changes in blood sugar levels.

A good diet and regular exercise are crucial for treating gestational diabetes in addition to monitoring blood sugar levels. A healthy diet reduced in sugar and carbohydrates can help control blood sugar levels. An individualized food plan for pregnant women with gestational diabetes may require collaboration with a qualified dietitian. Foods high in nutrients, such as lean protein, whole grains, fruits, and vegetables, should be included in a meal plan.

For women with gestational diabetes, exercise is a crucial component of self-care. Frequent exercise helps to enhance insulin sensitivity and blood sugar regulation.

A minimum of 30 minutes of moderate activity, such as brisk walking or swimming, should be performed by pregnant women with gestational diabetes each day. Before beginning an exercise regimen, women with gestational diabetes should consult their doctor to be sure it is safe for both them and their unborn child.

Another crucial component of self-care for pregnant diabetic women is stress management. Stress can impact blood sugar levels, and pregnancy can be a stressful period. Deep breathing exercises, yoga, meditation, or other relaxation methods may be helpful for pregnant women with gestational diabetes. A healthy lifestyle and stress management both depend on getting adequate sleep.

For women with gestational diabetes, proactive management is just as important as self-care. This entails going to prenatal checkups on time and according to the doctor's recommended course of action. To help control their blood sugar levels, women with gestational diabetes may need to take medicine or insulin. In order to make sure the treatment plan is successful; it is crucial to strictly adhere to the prescription schedule and check blood sugar levels.

In order to guarantee a healthy pregnancy and infant, women with gestational diabetes must practice self-care and proactive management. A good diet and exercise routine, stress management techniques, routine prenatal checkups, and routine blood sugar monitoring are all crucial components of self-care. To lower the risk of complications, women with gestational diabetes should closely collaborate with their healthcare professional to create a specific treatment plan and adhere to it religiously.

A Message for Pregnant Diabetic Women.

I want to provide a message of encouragement and hope to every woman who has been told she has gestational diabetes. When you get this news, it's normal to feel terrified or overwhelmed, but please know that you are not alone.

Although managing gestational diabetes during pregnancy may seem difficult, it is possible with the correct resources and assistance. It's crucial to keep in mind that gestational diabetes is a treatable condition, and that you may have a healthy pregnancy and deliver a healthy baby by managing your health and adhering to the advice of your healthcare team.

Please don't hesitate to ask for assistance and support as you proceed on this adventure. There are people out there who care about you and want to see you succeed, whether it's from your medical team, your loved ones, or a support group. Recall to prioritize your well-being, maintain a nutritious diet, engage in regular exercise, and track your blood sugar levels faithfully.

You are able to overcome any challenge that comes your way because you are powerful and tenacious. In the end, your devotion to maintaining your health and the health of your child will pay off, and you'll come out of it stronger than ever.

So, breathe deeply, keep a cheerful attitude, and trust that you can handle this. You are a wonderful mother who is doing everything in her ability to give her child the best chance at success. Keep up the good job and know that you and your child have a better future ahead of them.